Cardiac Diet Cookbook for Picky Eaters

35+ Tasty Heart-Healthy and Low Sodium Recipes

Disclaimer

By reading this disclaimer, you are accepting the terms of the disclaimer in full. If you disagree with this disclaimer, please do not read the book. The content in this book is provided for informational and educational purposes only.

This book is not intended to be a substitute for the original work of this diet plan. At most, this book is intended to be a beginner's supplement to the original work for this diet plan and never acts as a direct substitute. This book is an overview, review, and commentary on the facts of that diet plan.

All product names, diet plans, or names used in this book are for identification purposes only and are property of their respective owners. The use of these names does not imply endorsement. All other trademarks cited herein are the property of their respective owners.

None of the information in this book should be accepted as an independent medical or other professional advice.

The information in the books has been compiled from various sources that are deemed reliable. It has been analyzed and summarized to the best of the Author's ability, knowledge, and belief. However, the Author cannot guarantee the accuracy and thus should not be held liable for any errors.

You acknowledge and agree that the Author of this book will not be held liable for any damages, costs, expenses, resulting from the application of the information in this book, whether directly or indirectly. You acknowledge and agree that you assume all risk and responsibility for any action you undertake in response to the information in this book.

You acknowledge and agree that by continuing to read this book, you will (where applicable, appropriate, or necessary) consult a qualified medical professional on this information. The information in this book is not intended to be any sort of medical advice and should not be used in lieu of any medical advice by a licensed and qualified medical professional.

Always seek the advice of your physician or another qualified health provider with any issues or questions you might have regarding any sort of medical condition. Do not ever disregard any qualified professional medical advice or delay seeking that advice because of anything you have read in this book.

Table of Contents

Introduction

Did you know that nearly half of all adult Americans have cardiovascular disease?

Cardiovascular diseases remain to be one of the leading causes of death worldwide. As such, numerous studies have been conducted over the years to develop effective means of lowering the risk for heart issues and improving the health condition of those who already have heart problems.

One of these methods is through the adaptation of the cardiac diet, which is composed of the following elements:
- Fresh and brightly colored vegetables
- Fresh fruits
- Unrefined, whole grains
- Plant-based food products
- Lean cuts of meat
- Healthy fats
- Anti-inflammatory beverages

This cookbook contains a curated collection of heart-healthy recipes that are tasty, yet healthy and fun to make. In addition, a sample 7-day meal plan is included to help accelerate your adoption of the cardiac diet.

Sample Meal Plan for a Healthier Heart

To get you started, here is a 7-day sample meal plan based on the principles of the cardiac diet.

Take note that the recipes for items that have been marked with an asterisk (*) can be found in the later parts of this guide.

Day 1
- Breakfast
    - Wholegrain Cereal with Raisins
    - Soymilk

- Morning Snack
    - Banana Slices
    - Plain Water

- Lunch
    - Tomato and Basil Salad
    - Ginger Pumpkin Soup
    - Non-Fat Yoghurt
    - Lemon Water

- Afternoon Snack
    - Dried apricots
    - English Tea

- Dinner
    - Oriental-Style Salmon Fillet

- Apple and Onion Mix*
- Dry Red Wine

Day 2
- Breakfast
  - Banana Oatmeal Muffin
  - Green Tea

- Morning Snack
  - Fresh Fruit Cup
  - Plain Water

- Lunch
  - Shrimp & Egg Fried Rice*

- Afternoon Snack
  - Wholegrain Crackers
  - Hummus Dip
  - Water with Cucumber Slices

- Dinner
  - Chicken & Green Beans Stir-Fry
  - Greek Salad
  - Dry Red Wine

Day 3
- Breakfast
  - Toasted Bread with Honey
  - Strawberry Slices
  - Plain Water

- Morning Snack

- o Carrot Sticks
- o Green Smoothie

- Lunch
  - o Broccoli Mushroom Bisque
  - o Napa Cabbage Salad with Oriental Peanut Dressing
  - o Plain Water

- Afternoon Snack
  - o Banana Chips
  - o Plain Water

- Dinner
  - o Grilled Eggplant*
  - o Turkey Salad
  - o Dry Red Wine

Day 4
- Breakfast
  - o Honey-Sweetened Granola Bars
  - o English Tea

- Morning Snack
  - o Dried Mixed Berries
  - o Plain Water

- Lunch
  - o Pepper Ginger Beef Stir-Fry*
  - o Feta Fruit Salad
  - o Plain Water

- Afternoon Snack
  - Spinach and Kale Smoothie

- Dinner
  - Mushroom and Kale Casserole
  - Turkey and Black Bean Burgers
  - Dry Red Wine

Day 5
- Breakfast
  - Cherry Oatmeal
  - Toasted Whole Wheat Bread
  - Plain Water

- Morning Snack
  - Apple Slices
  - Lemon Water

- Lunch
  - Baked Eggplant Slices
  - Lettuce, Arugula, White Beans, And Tomato Salad with Italian Dressing
  - Plain Water

- Afternoon Snack
  - Mixed Berries Smoothie

- Dinner
  - Salmon & Asparagus*
  - Dry Red Wine

Day 6

- Breakfast
  - Chickpea Omelet with Onions and Mushroom
  - English Tea

- Morning Snack
  - Banana Bread*
  - English Tea

- Lunch
  - Taco Salad Wraps
  - Butternut Squash & Turmeric Soup*
  - Plain Water

- Afternoon Snack
  - Strawberry Slices
  - Plain Water

- Dinner
  - Mixed Greens and Orange Salad with Honey-Miso Dressing
  - Avocado and Cheese Sandwich
  - Dry Red Wine

Day 7
- Breakfast
  - Dark Chocolate Muffin
  - Ginger Tea

- Morning Snack
  - Blueberry Smoothie

- Lunch
  - Cheddar Turkey Deviled Egg *
  - Steamed Asparagus
  - Lemon Water

- Afternoon Snack
  - Melon Slices
  - Plain Water

- Dinner
  - Broccoli and Chickpea Salad
  - Baked Eggplant and Tomato Slices with Parmesan and Parsley
  - Dry Red Wine

Recipe List

Refer to the recipes below for suggested dishes that best exemplifies the principles of the cardiac diet.

Each has been carefully incorporated into the meal plan given earlier to give a background on the makings an ideal heart-friendly meal plan.

If you want to substitute any of the ingredients below, or if you think that there is a better way of cooking these dishes, then feel free to experiment, as long as you will remain within the confines of what is allowable in the cardiac diet. When in doubt, refer back to the cardiac diet food pyramid, and the various tips and suggestions given in the preceding chapters.

Apple and Onion Mix

Ingredients:

- ✓ 1 medium-sized Granny Smith apple, finely diced
- ✓ ¼ cup red onion, finely chopped
- ✓ ¼ cup walnuts, toasted, finely chopped
- ✓ 1 tablespoon extra-virgin olive oil OR walnut oil
- ✓ 1 teaspoon lemon juice
- ✓ 1 teaspoon honey
- ✓ ½ teaspoon sage, finely chopped
- ✓ A pinch of salt

Procedure:

1. Place apple dices, chopped onion, chopped walnuts, chopped sage, oil, honey, and lemon juice in a bowl.
2. Toss until all ingredients are evenly distributed and coated with honey-lemon dressing.
3. Sprinkle with salt to taste.
4. Serve immediately.

Yield: 1 to 2 servings

Shrimp and Egg Fried Rice

Ingredients:

- ✓ ¾ cup long-grained jasmine rice washed
- ✓ ½ cup of water
- ✓ 1 cup chicken broth, no salt
- ✓ 4 ounces large shrimps (around 35 pieces per pound), peeled and deveined, sliced into ½-inch bits, patted dry
- ✓ 2 large eggs, beaten
- ✓ 2 cups sugar snap peas, trimmed and cut into two
- ✓ 1 cup shiitake mushrooms, caps only
- ✓ 1 cup carrots, diced into 1/4-inch bits
- ✓ 2 tablespoons low-sodium soy sauce
- ✓ 1 tablespoon garlic, minced
- ✓ 1 tablespoon fresh ginger, minced
- ✓ ¼ teaspoon red chili pepper, crushed
- ✓ 2 tablespoons vegetable oil

✓ 1/8 teaspoon ground white pepper

Procedure:

1. Combine and boil the chicken broth and water into a small saucepan.
2. Add washed jasmine rice.
3. Reduce the heat to low.
4. Cover the saucepan with its lid.
5. Simmer until the rice has become tender, and the liquid has vaporized.
6. Remove from heat.
7. In a frying pan, heat the vegetable oil for half a minute.
8. Add minced garlic, minced ginger, and crushed red chili peppers.
9. Stir fry using a metal spatula for about 10 seconds, or until mixture has become fragrant.
10. Add diced carrots and mushroom caps.
11. Stir fry for about 1 minute.
12. Add shrimp slices.
13. Stir fry for another minute.
14. Add sugar snap pear halves.
15. Stir fry for 1 minute, or until peas have turned bright green.
16. Remove from heat.

17. Add beaten eggs, cooked rice, soy sauce, and pepper.

18. While still off the heat, stir fry for about 1 to minutes, or until shrimp are cooked through and the eggs have set.

19. Transfer into a bowl and serve while it is still hot.

Yield: 2 to 3 servings

Grilled Eggplant

Ingredients:

- ✓ 2 small eggplants OR 1 large eggplant

- ✓ 2 tablespoons extra-virgin olive oil

- ✓ A pinch of salt

Procedure:

1. Pre-heat the grill using the medium-high setting.

2. Toss eggplant slices and olive oil in a bowl.

3. Sprinkle with salt to taste.

4. Toss the ingredients again.

5. Place eggplant slices into the grill.

6. Turn over to the other side after about 4 minutes, or until charred spots have appeared on the underside.

7. Continue grilling until eggplant slices have become tender.

Yield: 2 servings

Tip: You can prepare this dish ahead of time. Just place into an airtight container once it has cooled down, and then refrigerate. Grilled eggplant can last for up to 4 days in chilled condition.

Mixed Vegetable Roast with Lemon Zest

Ingredients:

- ✓ 1½ cups broccoli florets
- ✓ 1½ cups cauliflower florets
- ✓ ¾ cup red bell pepper, diced by 1-inch cuts
- ✓ ¾ cup zucchini, diced by 1-inch cuts
- ✓ 2 thinly sliced cloves of garlic
- ✓ lemon zest (2 teaspoons)
- ✓ olive oil (1 tablespoon)
- ✓ A pinch of salt
- ✓ 1 teaspoon dried and crushed oregano

Procedure:

1. Preheat oven set to 425°F.

2. Combine garlic and both florets (broccoli and cauliflower) in a baking pan (15-by-10-inch). Drizzle oil over the vegetables and sprinkle with salt

and oregano; stir long enough to coat. Roast for 10 minutes.

3. Add zucchini and bell pepper to the rest of the mix in the pan; toss to combine. Continue roasting for 10 to 15 minutes more until the pieces are lightly browned and are crisp-tender.

4. Before serving, drizzle lemon zest over the vegetables and toss.

Yield: 1 to 2 servings

Pepper Ginger Beef Stir-Fry

Ingredients:

- ✓ 6 ounces (175 grams) lean rump OR fillet steak, thinly cut into strips across the grain

- ✓ 2 ounces (55 grams) mange tout, trimmed

- ✓ 4 spring onions, chopped

- ✓ 1 small red bell pepper, deseeded and thinly cut into strips

- ✓ 1 small green OR yellow bell pepper, deseeded and thinly cut into strips

- ✓ 1 ½ teaspoon Sichuan pepper, crushed

- ✓ 1 fresh red chili, deseeded and finely chopped

- ✓ 1 carrot, cut into thin sticks

- ✓ 0.8-inch (2-cm) fresh ginger, peeled and thinly cut into strips

- ✓ 1 clove garlic, finely chopped

- ✓ A dash of low-sodium soy sauce

- ✓ 4 tablespoons water
- ✓ 2-3 teaspoons sunflower oil
- ✓ 1 teaspoon cornflour
- ✓ 1 teaspoon soft dark brown sugar

Procedure:

1. Mix cornflour and water in a small bowl until the texture has become smooth.

2. Stir in soy sauce and sugar until the particles have been completely dissolved. Set aside.

3. In a non-stick wok, heat 1 teaspoon of sunflower oil using the medium setting of the stove.

4. Add the beef strips and crushed pepper.

5. Stir-fry for about 3 to 4 minutes, or until the beef strips have turned brown.

6. Transfer the beef strips into a plate using a slotted spoon. Set aside.

7. Pour the remaining sunflower oil into the work.

8. Heat the oil using the medium setting.

9. Add the garlic, red chili, mange tout, peppers, carrot, spring onions, and ginger into the wok.

10. Stir-fry for 3 to 5 minutes or until preferred texture is achieved.

11. Return the stir-fried beef strips from earlier.

12. Pour the cornflour mixture into the can

13. Stir fry for 1 to minutes, or until beef strips have become hot again.

14. Serve immediately over cooked rice or rice noodles.

Yield: 2 to 3 servings

Salmon and Asparagus

Ingredients:

- ✓ 2 salmon fillets, around 5 ounces
- ✓ 14 ounces (397 grams) young potatoes
- ✓ 8 asparagus spears, trimmed and halved
- ✓ 2 handfuls cherry tomatoes
- ✓ 1 handful basil leaves
- ✓ 2 tablespoons extra-virgin olive oil
- ✓ 1 tablespoon balsamic vinegar

Procedure:

1. Heat oven to 428 °F

2. Arrange the potatoes into a baking dish.

3. Drizzle potatoes with 1 tablespoon extra-virgin olive oil.

4. Roast potatoes for 20 minutes, or until they have turned golden brown.

5. Place the asparagus into the baking dish together with the potatoes.

6. Roast in the oven for another 15 minutes.

7. Arrange the cherry tomatoes and salmon among the vegetables.

8. Drizzle with balsamic vinegar and the remaining olive oil.

9. Roast for 10 to 15 minutes, or until salmon is cooked.

10. Throw in a handful of basil leaves before transferring everything in a serving dish.

11. Serve while hot.

Yield: 2 servings

Baked Salmon

Ingredients

- ✓ 1 1/4 lb Salmon—King, Sockeye or Coho salmon
- ✓ 1/4 tsp black pepper—to taste
- ✓ 3 cloves garlic, minced—or 1 tsp garlic powder
- ✓ 1 tbsp fresh chopped dill
- ✓ 2 tbsp olive oil
- ✓ 1 tbsp lemon juice

Directions

1. Preheat oven to 350F. Grease a sheet pan of a porcelain baking dish with olive oil. Season salmon on both sides with salt and pepper.
2. In a small bowl combine the rest of the olive oil, garlic, dill, lemon juice. Place salmon skin side down in the baking dish. Pour the mixture over the salmon and spread on top.
3. Bake for 15-20 minutes, until the fish is no longer opaque on top.
4. If you'd like it to look golden on top, broil for 1 minute, (425F) keeping an eye on it. Thermometer inserted in the middle should read 145 F.

5. Garnish with fresh dill and lemon slices. Serve.

Roasted Veggies

Ingredients:

- ✓ ½ pound turnips
- ✓ ½ lb. carrots
- ✓ ½ lb. parsnips
- ✓ 2 medium-sized shallots, peeled
- ✓ ¼ tsp ground black pepper
- ✓ 2 tbsps. extra-virgin olive oil
- ✓ 6 cloves garlic (with skin)
- ✓ 2 tbsps. fresh rosemary needles

Directions:

1. First cut vegetables into bite sized pieces (or your chosen size)
2. Set the oven to 400°F.
3. Mix all the ingredients in a 9x13-inch baking dish.
2. Roast the vegetables for 25 minutes until brown and tender.
3. Toss and roast again for 20- 25 minutes.
4. Then serve hot.

Trout Scrambler

Instructions

- ✓ 1 small potato, cut into 8 wedges
- ✓ ½ tsp extra-virgin olive oil
- ✓ Freshly ground black pepper to taste
- ✓ 1 cup spinach
- ✓ 1 egg, scrambled
- ✓ 3 ounces trout fillet
- ✓ Dash of salt

Instructions

1. Preheat oven to 375°F. Toss potatoes, ⅛ tsp of olive oil, and black pepper. Place on a sheet tray and bake until the potatoes are tender approximately 10 minutes.
2. Remove from oven, toss in spinach, and set aside.
3. Heat 2 heavy-bottomed skillets over low heat. In a small bowl, combine the egg and black pepper. Put ⅛ tsp of olive oil in one pan, pour in the egg, and cook, stirring constantly until it reaches your desired doneness.

4. Place ⅛ tsp of olive oil in the second pan and cook the fish until slightly browned approximately 3 minutes. Flip and cook until the fish are just beginning to flake but the center is still translucent 2 minutes.
5. Serve the spinach and potato mixture with the scrambled egg and fish. Just before eating, season the eggs and fish with a dash of salt

Cod Pea Curry

Instructions

- ✓ 1 tbsp extra-virgin olive oil
- ✓ 1 onion, sliced
- ✓ 1 tsp cumin
- ✓ 1 tsp mustard powder
- ✓ ½ tsp turmeric
- ✓ 1 tbsp minced fresh ginger
- ✓ 1 tsp minced garlic
- ✓ A pinch of salt
- ✓ Freshly ground black pepper
- ✓ Pinch of cayenne, or to taste
- ✓ 2 cups chopped tomatoes
- ✓ 2 tbsp. finely chopped cilantro
- ✓ 1 medium head cauliflower, broken into small florets, approximately half-inch pieces
- ✓ 1-pound cod, cut into cubes, about half an inch each
- ✓ 2 cups fresh or frozen peas
- ✓ 4 cups spinach

Instructions

1. Heat a large heavy-bottomed stockpot over low heat. Add the olive oil and onion and cook until

translucent, stirring often, 5 minutes. Add the cumin, mustard powder, turmeric, ginger, garlic, salt, black pepper, and cayenne. Cook for 1 more minute, stirring constantly.

2. Add the tomatoes, cilantro, and 4½ cups of water. Bring to a boil, reduce to a simmer, and cook for 10 minutes.

3. Add the cauliflower; return to a simmer and cook for 2 minutes. Add the cod, peas, and spinach; stir and cover. Simmer for 4 minutes and serve immediately

Mixed Veggie Fried Rice

Ingredients:

- ✓ 2 tablespoons of minced garlic
- ✓ 2 eggs, beaten
- ✓ ¼ cup of minced carrots and onions
- ✓ ½ cup of chopped tomatoes
- ✓ 1/8 cup of chopped parsley
- ✓ a cup of brown rice
- ✓ ¼ teaspoon of white ground pepper
- ✓ ¼ teaspoon salt
- ✓ 1/8 teaspoon of ground turmeric for added flavor

Procedure:

Cook the rice and eggs separately. Once you have cooked the eggs, slice them into thin strips.
Pour olive or canola oil into the skillet. Toss in the cooked brown rice. Add the rest of the ingredients. Sprinkle ground turmeric. You may also add half a teaspoon of balsamic vinegar, though this is optional.

Arugula and Mushroom Salad

Ingredients:

- ✓ 5 oz. arugula washed
- ✓ 1 lb. fresh mushrooms
- ✓ ¼ teaspoon shoyu
- ✓ ½ red onion
- ✓ Tofu cheese*
- ✓ 1 tablespoon olive oil
- ✓ 1 tablespoon mirin

Tofu Cheese Ingredients:
- ✓ ⅛ cup umeboshi vinegar
- ✓ ½ firm tofu

Instructions:

1. In a small bowl, add the rinsed tofu; crumble and pour in the vinegar.
2. In a medium-sized bowl add the shoyu, tofu cheese, red onions, salt, olive oil, and mirin; mix to combine.
3. Add in the arugula and toss to combine with the dressing.
4. Serve on a plate

Cyprian Cheese and Greens Salad with Pesto Dressing

Ingredients:

Salad
- ✓ 2 heads lettuce (large)
- ✓ 1/4 bulb fennel
- ✓ 2 cucumbers
- ✓ 1 avocado
- ✓ ¼ cup toasted almonds
- ✓ 1 packet halloumi/vegan cheese
- ✓ ¼ cup basil leaves
- ✓ 1/8 cup dill
- ✓ Black peppercorns
- ✓ 2 tablespoon lemon juice
- ✓ Olive oil

Pesto Sauce:
- ✓ 1 cup toasted almonds
- ✓ 1 lemon
- ✓ 1/2 cup arugula
- ✓ 1 cup olive oil

Instructions:

1. In a food processor, prepare the pesto sauce by adding all ingredients together; blend to smoothen; season with lemon juice, pepper, and salt to taste.

2. In a large salad bowl, add the herbs and remaining vegetables.
3. Transfer pesto sauce in a small bowl, and serve with the salad.
4. In a pan, prepare the halloumi by frying until crunchy at the sides; serve salad greens and pesto sauce.

Macrobiotic Bowl Medley

Ingredients:

For the Bowl
- ✓ 1/2 cup brown rice
- ✓ 3 cup chard, roughly chopped
- ✓ 1 cup squash, diced
- ✓ 1 cup broccoli florets
- ✓ 1 cup black beans
- ✓ 1 oz. kombu
- ✓ 1/2 cup sauerkraut, chopped

For the Sauce
- ✓ 2 tablespoon sesame tahini
- ✓ 2 tablespoon sodium tamari
- ✓ 1 clove garlic
- ✓ 1 tablespoon ginger
- ✓ 1 lime, juiced

Instructions:

For the Bowl
1. Bring 1 cup of water to a boil for the rice. Once boiling, add rice, return to boil, cover then reduce heat and simmer 40 minutes. Remove from heat and allow to sit covered an additional 10 minutes then fluff with a fork.

2. Thoroughly rinse and drain beans, then transfer to a pot with kombu, cover with water, bring to a boil, reduce heat and simmer 15-20 minutes then drain and rinse.
3. Place a steamer basket in a pot with water and bring to a boil.
4. Add broccoli, cover and steam 4-5 minutes then remove, keeping water in the pot.
5. Add squash, cover and steam 4-5 minutes then remove, keeping water in the pot.
6. Add chard, cover and steam 3-4 minutes, then remove.

Broccoli-Kale with Avocado Toppings Rice Bowl

Ingredients:

- ✓ 1/2 avocado
- ✓ 2 cups kale
- ✓ 1 cup broccoli florets
- ✓ 1/2 cup cooked brown rice
- ✓ 1 teaspoon plum vinegar
- ✓ 2 teaspoon tamari
- ✓ Sea salt, to taste

Instructions:

1. In a small pot, simmer broccoli florets, and kale in about 3 tablespoons of water; cook for 2 minutes.
2. Add tamari, vinegar, and cooked brown rice; stir to combine.
3. Transfer pot contents into a medium-sized bowl and top with sliced avocado; sprinkle a dash of sea salt to taste.

Stir Fry Broccoli, Onions and Carrots

Ingredients:

- ✓ 1 teaspoon light olive oil
- ✓ 1 ½ cups onion
- ✓ 2 cups medium-sized carrots
- ✓ 6 cups medium-sized broccoli
- ✓ 2 ½-inch broccoli flowerets
- ✓ ¼ teaspoon of sea salt
- ✓ ½ cup of water
- ✓ 1 tablespoon soy sauce (optional)

Instructions:

1. In a pan, heat the sesame oil to medium-high heat; add to sauté the onions.
2. Sauté the carrots, broccoli, the flowerets, then add water; season with sea salt and cover the pan to bring to a boil.
3. Lower the heat and bring to a simmer for 5 minutes.
4. Pour some soy sauce if needed.

Reminder:

1. Stir-fried vegetables, top with some pasta or rice.

2. Substitute other vegetables such as cabbage, cabbage, cauliflower, or yellow squash.
3. For additional flavor, sauté 1 tablespoon of minced ginger in the oil before adding the carrots.

Banana Bread

Ingredients:

- ✓ 10.6 ounces (300 grams) overripe bananas, mashed

- ✓ 5 ounces (140 grams) whole-wheat flour

- ✓ 3.5 ounces (100 grams) self-rising flour

- ✓ 3 large eggs, beaten

- ✓ 10 tablespoons natural, low-fat yogurt

- ✓ 4 tablespoons agave syrup

- ✓ 1 teaspoon sodium bicarbonate

- ✓ 1 teaspoon baking powder

- ✓ 0.88-ounce (25 grams) pecan OR walnuts, chopped

- ✓ low-fat butter spread

Procedure:

1. Heat the oven to 320 °F (160 °C or gas 3 settings).

2. Grease a 2-pound loaf tin before lining it with baking parchment that is at least 1 inch over the top edges.

3. Mix the whole-wheat flour, self-rising flour, sodium bicarbonate, baking powder, and a pinch of salt in a large bowl.

4. Mix the bananas, agave syrup, eggs, and yogurt in a separate bowl.

5. Quickly stir in the wet ingredients into dry ingredients.

6. Gently scrape the batter into the tin.

7. Scatter with chopped nuts on top, if you are using them.

8. Bake for 1 hour-10 min up to 1 hour-15 min, or until a cake tester or skewer comes out clean.

9. Cooldown the bread while it is still in the tin on a wire rack.

10. Serve warm or at ambient temperature, with low-fat spread on the side.

Yield: 6 to 8 servings

Butternut Squash and Turmeric Soup

Ingredients:

- ✓ 1 medium butternut squash (about 2 ½ lbs.), peeled and chopped into 1-inch pieces, reserve the seeds

- ✓ 2 medium carrots, cut into 1-inch pieces

- ✓ 2 ¼ teaspoon turmeric powder

- ✓ 1 large onion, roughly chopped

- ✓ 2 tablespoons light coconut milk

- ✓ 1 tablespoon vegetable soup base OR 1 vegetable bouillon cube

- ✓ 2 ½ tablespoons extra-virgin olive oil

- ✓ 2 ¼ teaspoon ground black pepper

Procedure:

1. Heat 2 tablespoons of oil in a large Dutch oven (cast-iron pot) using medium heat.

2. Add the onion and cover the pot with its lid.

3. Cook, while stirring occasionally, for 6 to 8 minutes, or until onions have become tender.

4. Mix the soup base or bouillon with 6 cups of boiling water.

5. Stir until all powder or cube has been dissolved.

6. Add the carrots, squash, 2 teaspoons of turmeric, and ½ teaspoon of ground black pepper into the pot.

7. Cook for 1 minute while stirring occasionally.

8. Pour the soup broth into the pot.

9. Bring to a boil before reducing the heat.

10. Simmer for 18 to 22 minutes, or until vegetables have become very tender.

11. Heat oven to 375°F (191 ºC).

12. Toss ¼ cup of the reserved seeds with the remaining oil, ¼ teaspoon turmeric, and ¼ teaspoon black pepper.

13. Roast for about 9 to 11 minutes, or until seeds have become crispy and golden brown

14. Puree the soup using an immersion blender.

15. Sprinkle with toasted seeds on top, and swirl in the coconut milk.

16. Serve immediately.

Yield: 3 to 4 servings

Cheddar Turkey Deviled Egg

Ingredients:

- ✓ 6 large organic eggs
- ✓ 2 slices nitrate-free turkey bacon
- ✓ ¼ cup low-fat cheddar cheese, shredded OR grated
- ✓ 3 tablespoons light mayonnaise
- ✓ 1 teaspoon white wine vinegar
- ✓ ½ teaspoon chives, chopped
- ✓ 1/8 teaspoon ground black pepper
- ✓ 1/8 teaspoon salt

Procedure:

1. Place the eggs in a large pot or saucepan.
2. Pour cold water into the pot or pan until the water is covering the eggs by 1 ½ inches.
3. Bring the water to a boil over high heat.
4. Once it has boiled, remove the pot, or pan from the stove.

5. Cover the pot or pan, and let it stand for 12 to 15 minutes.

6. When it has cooled down, peel off the egg's shells.

7. Fry the bacon slices using medium-high heat in a non-stick skillet until bacon slices have become crispy but not burnt.

8. Transfer fried bacon into paper towels to drain off the excess oil.

9. Once it has cooled down, break down the bacon into small bits. Set aside.

10. Cut the hard-boiled eggs into half, lengthwise.

11. Gently carve out the egg yolks into a medium-sized bowl.

12. Arrange the hollowed-out egg halves in a flat container.

13. Add the rest of the ingredients into the bowl with the yolk.

14. Stir well until the texture has become smooth.

15. Transfer the mixture into a piping bag or resealable bag with a trimmed corner.

16. Pipe the yolk mixture back into the egg halves.

17. Sprinkle each filled egg halves with bacon bits.

18. Serve immediately or after it has been chilled for at least half an hour.

Yield: 3 to 4 servings

Go Green Blueberries

Ingredients:
- ✓ 2 cups chopped spinach
- ✓ 1/4 cup water
- ✓ 1/3 cup chopped carrot
- ✓ 1/2 cup blueberries
- ✓ 1/2 cup chopped cucumber
- ✓ 1/4 cup almond milk
- ✓ 4 ice cubes

Procedure:
1. Using a blender, mix the water and spinach. Slowly turn up the speed until no solid particles are present.
2. After the mixture has homogenized, add the other ingredients.
3. Continue to increase speed until you reach the maximum speed for 30 seconds.
4. Serve chilled.

Yield: 2

Spinach and Kale blend

Ingredients:
- ✓ 1 cup spinach
- ✓ 1 cup chopped kale
- ✓ 3/4 cup water
- ✓ 1/2 cup chopped cucumber
- ✓ 1 green apple
- ✓ 1 cup chopped papaya
- ✓ 1 tablespoon ground flaxseed

Procedure:
1. Using a blender, mix the water, spinach, and kale. Increase speed until all solid particles are gone.
2. Add the rest of the ingredients. Resume blending until reaching the maximum speed.
3. Maintain the maximum speed for 30 seconds before serving.
4. Serve chilled.

Yield: 2

Energy Boost Smoothie

Ingredients:
- ✓ 1 large rib celery
- ✓ 1 tablespoon parsley
- ✓ 3/4 cup water
- ✓ 1/2 cup chopped cooked beets
- ✓ 1 small orange, segmented
- ✓ 3/4 cup chopped carrot

Procedure:
1. Using a blender, mix the water, parsley, and celery. Increase speed until all solid particles are gone.
2. Add the rest of the ingredients. Resume blending until reaching the maximum speed.
3. Maintain the maximum speed for 30 seconds before serving.
4. Serve chilled.

Yield: 2

Green and Berry Smoothie

Ingredients:
- ✓ 2 cups spinach
- ✓ 2 large kale leaves
- ✓ 3/4 cup water
- ✓ 1 large frozen banana
- ✓ 1/2 cup frozen mango
- ✓ 1/2 cup frozen peach
- ✓ 1 tablespoon ground flaxseeds
- ✓ 1 tablespoon almond butter or peanut butter

Procedure:
1. Using a blender, mix the water, spinach, and kale. Increase speed until all solid particles are gone.
2. Add the rest of the ingredients. Resume blending until reaching the maximum speed.
3. Maintain the maximum speed for 30 seconds before serving.
4. Serve chilled.

Yield: 2

Almond Surf Smoothie

Ingredients:
- ✓ 1 large banana
- ✓ 1 cup almond milk
- ✓ 1 tablespoon almond butter
- ✓ 1 tablespoon wheat germ
- ✓ 1/8 teaspoon vanilla extract
- ✓ 1/8 teaspoon ground cinnamon
- ✓ 3–4 ice cubes

Procedure:
1. Using a blender, place all the ingredients and start blending.
2. Increase speed until you reach the intermediate speed setting.
3. Maintain speed for 30 seconds before serving.
4. Serve chilled.

Yield: 1

- Toasted Almond Banana Mix

Ingredients:
- ✓ 2 slices whole-wheat bread
- ✓ 2 tablespoons almond butter
- ✓ 1 small banana
- ✓ 1/8 teaspoon ground cinnamon

Procedure:

1. Start by toasting each piece of bread.
2. After toasting, add the butter.
3. Add the banana slices and a pinch of cinnamon.
4. Serve Immediately.

Yield: 1

- Berry Blast English Muffin

Ingredients:
- ✓ 1 English muffin, halved
- ✓ 1 tablespoon cream cheese
- ✓ 4 strawberries
- ✓ 1/2 cup blueberries

Procedure:
1. Start by toasting each half of the muffin.
2. After being toasted, add the cream cheese on each half.
3. Add the berries.
4. Serve immediately.

Yield: 1

Berry Blast Oats

Ingredients:
- ✓ 1 1/2 cups plain almond milk
- ✓ 1/8 teaspoon vanilla extract
- ✓ 1 cup oats
- ✓ 3/4 cup mix of blueberries and blackberries
- ✓ 2 tablespoons toasted pecans

Procedure:
1. With a small frying pan, warm up the vanilla and almond milk together using medium fire.
2. Right before the ingredients boil, add the oat. Cook for 5 minutes.
3. Add the berries.
4. Serve hot.

Yield: 2

- Apple Cinnamon Smash Oatmeal

Ingredients:
- ✓ 1 1/2 cups plain almond milk
- ✓ 1 cup oats
- ✓ 1 large Granny Smith apple
- ✓ 1/4 teaspoon ground cinnamon
- ✓ 2 tablespoons toasted walnut pieces

Procedure:

1. Heat the apple and oats together in low to medium fire.
2. Continue heating for 5 minutes.
3. Add the cinnamon.
4. Serve hot.

Yield: 2

Energizing Oatmeal

Ingredients:
- ✓ 1/4 cup water
- ✓ 1/4 cup milk
- ✓ 1/2 cup oats
- ✓ 4 egg whites
- ✓ 1/8 teaspoon ground cinnamon
- ✓ 1/8 teaspoon ground ginger
- ✓ 1/4 cup blueberries

Procedure:
1. Start by mixing the milk and water in a pan.
2. Heat the mixture on the stove using medium settings.
3. Just before the mixture boils, add the oats and continue heating for 5 minutes.
4. Mix in the whites, continue cooking for 4 minutes.
5. Add the ginger and cinnamon.
6. Serve hot.

Yield: 1

Quinoa-based Oriental Salad

Ingredients:
- ✓ 2 cups uncooked quinoa
- ✓ 4 cups vegetable broth
- ✓ 1 cup edamame
- ✓ 1/4 cup chopped green onion
- ✓ 1 1/2 teaspoons chopped fresh mint
- ✓ 1/2 cup chopped carrot
- ✓ 1/2 cup chopped red bell pepper
- ✓ 1/8 teaspoon pepper flakes
- ✓ 1/2 teaspoon grated orange zest
- ✓ 2 tablespoons chopped fresh Thai basil
- ✓ Juice from half an orange
- ✓ 1 teaspoon sesame seeds
- ✓ 1 tablespoon sesame oil
- ✓ 1 tablespoon olive oil
- ✓ 1/8 teaspoon black pepper

Procedure:
1. Mix the broth and quinoa in a pan.
2. Set the stove to high and place the pan. Let the mixture heat up for 12 to 14 minutes.
3. After heating, cover the pan and wait for 4 minutes.
4. Place the mixture in a separate container and add the rest of the ingredients.
5. Let it cool down before serving.

Yield: 6

Hearty Chicken Salad with Pasta

Ingredients:
- ✓ 8 ounces penne pasta
- ✓ 1 (6-ounce) chicken breast
- ✓ 1 cup seedless red grapes
- ✓ 1/4 cup walnut pieces
- ✓ 1 tablespoon red wine vinegar
- ✓ 1/2 cup chopped celery
- ✓ 1/2 cup Greek yogurt
- ✓ 1/2 teaspoon black pepper
- ✓ 1/8 teaspoon salt

Procedure:
1. Start by cooking the pasta, a small addition of cooking oil is recommended.
2. Continue cooking the pasta for 7 – 9 minutes before removing the water.
3. Remove the fat off the chicken and chop it into small pieces.
4. Boil some water and place the chopped chicken into it. Boil for 7 minutes.
5. Remove water from both ingredients.
6. Add both the chicken and pasta together with the rest of the ingredients.
7. Cooldown before serving.

Yield: 6

Heart Helping Cobb

Ingredients:
- ✓ 4 slices turkey bacon
- ✓ 5 cups spinach
- ✓ 1 cup sliced cremini mushrooms
- ✓ 1/2 cup shredded carrot
- ✓ 1/2 cucumber
- ✓ 1/2 (15-ounce) can kidney beans
- ✓ 1 large avocado
- ✓ 1/3 cup crumbled blue cheese

Procedure:
1. Coat your frying pan with oil.
2. Place the bacon and turkey. Cook for 7 minutes.
3. Cut both bacon and turkey into small pieces.
4. Arrange on the plate with the rest of the ingredients.
5. Serve hot.

Yield: 4

Grenade Salad

Ingredients:
- ✓ 4 cups arugula
- ✓ 1 large avocado
- ✓ 1/2 cup sliced fennel
- ✓ 1/2 cup sliced Anjou pears
- ✓ 1/4 cup pomegranate seeds

Procedure:
1. Add together all the ingredients aside from the pomegranate seeds.
2. After mixing well, add the seeds and mix well.
3. Serve with any type of desired dressing.

Yield: 4

Chicken Breast Delight

Ingredients:
- ✓ 1 teaspoon dried oregano
- ✓ 1/2 teaspoon rosemary
- ✓ 1/2 teaspoon garlic powder
- ✓ 1/8 teaspoon salt
- ✓ Finely ground Black pepper
- ✓ 4 chicken breasts

Procedure:
1. Remove any fat from the breasts.
2. Mix the remaining ingredients in a separate container.
3. Add the mixture on either side of the chicken.
4. Prepare a frying pan, lightly oil the pan, and set the stove to medium.
5. Add the chicken into the frying pan. Cook for 3 to 5 minutes on each face.
6. Cool the chicken for a couple of minutes after cooking.
7. Serve warm.

Yield: 4

Sun Crust Turkey Cuts

Ingredients:
- ✓ 2 (6-ounce) turkey breasts
- ✓ 1 1/2 cups sunflower seeds
- ✓ 1/4 teaspoon ground cumin
- ✓ 2 tablespoons chopped parsley
- ✓ 1/4 teaspoon paprika
- ✓ 1/4 teaspoon cayenne pepper
- ✓ 1/4 teaspoon black pepper
- ✓ 1/3 cup whole wheat flour
- ✓ 3 egg whites

Procedure:
1. Start by warming up the oven to around 395 degrees F.
2. Prepare the breasts by cutting it into ¼ inch thick slices.
3. Mix the parsley, paprika, cumin, cayenne, sunflower seeds, and pepper in a processor.
4. Prepare the whites and flour in a separate container each.
5. Coat each breast part with the mixtures separately starting with the flour mixture, proceeding to the whites and then the processed mixture.
6. After coating all breasts, prepare the pan.
7. Bake the breasts for approximately 12 minutes on the oven.

8. Flip each side and resume baking for another 12 minutes.
9. Serve hot.

Yield: 4

Turkish Meatballs in Marinara

Ingredients:
- ✓ 1-pound ground turkey
- ✓ 1/2 small onion
- ✓ 2 large cloves garlic,
- ✓ 1/4 cup red bell pepper
- ✓ 3 tablespoons chopped parsley
- ✓ 1/2 teaspoon pepper flakes
- ✓ 1/8 teaspoon ground cumin
- ✓ 1/2 teaspoon dried Pre-mixed Italian herbs
- ✓ 1/8 teaspoon black pepper
- ✓ 1 egg
- ✓ 1/4 cup breadcrumbs
- ✓ 1/8 teaspoon salt
- ✓ 4 tablespoons olive oil
- ✓ 1 (16-ounce) jar marinara sauce
- ✓ 1/2 cup feta cheese

Procedure:
1. Start by warming the oven to 370F.
2. In a large container, mix most of the ingredients aside from the cheese, oil, and marinara.
3. Mix well and create the meatballs.
4. Open the stove at medium settings and prepare a frying pan.
5. Start searing the meatballs.

6. Once done with the meatballs. Prepare an oven pan.
7. Pace the meatballs along with the marinara together.
8. Bake for 20 – 30 minutes.
9. Serve hot.

Yield: 16 meatballs

Hot, Hot, Hot Salmon

Ingredients:
- ✓ 2 teaspoons chili powder
- ✓ 1 teaspoon ground cumin
- ✓ 1 teaspoon molasses
- ✓ 1/8 teaspoon salt
- ✓ 1/8 teaspoon black pepper
- ✓ 4 (4-ounce) salmon fillets
- ✓ Orange from half of an orange
- ✓ 2 tablespoons olive oil

Procedure:
1. Mix the pepper, sugar, chili powder, cumin, and salt.
2. Sprinkle the mixture onto the salmon.
3. Prepare a frying pan and set the stove to medium settings.
4. Add the salmon into the frying pan once hot. Cook for approximately 2 minutes.
5. Add the orange juice after 2 minutes on each face of the fillet.
6. Continue cooking for 3 more minutes.
7. Serve hot.

Yield: 4

Taste of Mediterranean

Ingredients:
- ✓ 1 cup uncooked couscous
- ✓ 1 1/4 cups water
- ✓ 1 (16-ounce) can artichoke hearts
- ✓ 1/2 cup kalamata olives
- ✓ 1 (12-ounce) jar roasted red pepper
- ✓ 1/2 cup feta cheese
- ✓ 1 cup cherry tomatoes
- ✓ 1/2 small onion
- ✓ 1/4 teaspoon chopped oregano
- ✓ 1/4 teaspoon chopped fresh mint
- ✓ ½ teaspoon Pepper flakes
- ✓ 4 tablespoons extra virgin olive oil
- ✓ Lemon Juice from a Single Lemon
- ✓ A piece of Black Pepper

Procedure:
1. Start by boiling water and adding the couscous. Mix well.
2. Turn off the stove after mixing.
3. Cover the mixture and cool for 6 minutes.
4. In a separate container, combine the rest of the ingredients.
5. Place the mixture in the fridge for 17 minutes.
6. Mix the mixture with the couscous.
7. Serve chilled.

Yield: 4

Conclusion

Thank you again for getting this cookbook.

If you found this cookbook helpful, please take the time to share your thoughts and post a review.

It would be greatly appreciated!

Thank you and good luck!